BOOST YOUR IMMUNE SYSTEM WITH DR SEBI APPROACH

•••Food and health via Dr Sebi approach.

(Brenda S. Hardin)

Table of

Contents

Table of Contents...2

CHAPTER ONE 8

WHO DR SEBI WAS 8

CHAPTER TWO 11

WHAT IS THE IMMUNE SYSTEM..........11

CLASSES OF FOOD THAT BOOST THE IMMUNE SYSTEM 16

WHAT DR. SEBI SAID ABOUT IMMUNITY 17

CHAPTER THREE 22

ANTI-OXIDANTS AND ANTI-INFLAMMATORY 22

OMEGA -3 FATTY ACIDS, FLAVONOIDS, AND MINERALS 27

CONCLUSION 60

Dedication

I dedicate this book to you for sacrificing your time and resources in pursuit of knowledge towards a healthier lifestyle.

INTRODUCTION

The importance of the immune system to the human body cannot be overemphasised as without the immune system the body is like a goal post without a keeper open to all kind of attack without a means of defence. A healthy immune system helps to protect the body against all forms of diseases or infections which threatens to pull down the systems of the body. Ten organs of the immune system stand as soldiers that fight these infections as keep the body healthy. To achieve these statuses of immune healthiness, we must feed on balanced and highly nutritious food. There are some foods whose primary purpose is to contribute actively to boosting the immune system and keeping it healthy to adequately perform its functions. These food are either gotten through natural processes, synthesized by the body or both. Both they work singly or collaboratively to enhance the activities of the immune system, maintain the health of immune organs, assist in proliferation, differentiation and all other activities that contribute towards body health. In this book, the activity, benefits and meal tips of each class of immune booster will be simplified and elaboratively explained for proper comprehension. Happy reading.

CHAPTER ONE

WHO DR SEBI WAS

The name Dr Sebi was an alias for a man named Alfredo Darrington Bowman. He was a Honduran herbalist (i.e. orthodox medicine practitioner) and a self-proclaimed healer, who claimed to have developed a unique approach and methodology to the healing of a human body irrespective of the disease with the sole use of herbs and food supplements. He was known to practice his form of medicine in the United States between the late 20th and early 21st century. He was recorded to be born on 26th of November, 1933 to Clifford Bowman and Violet Francis Bowman in Illanga, Honduras and died 6th of August 2016 in La Ceiba, Honduras. He was married to Patsy Bowman and Maha Bowman and was survived by 17 children Dr Sebi is of the firm belief that diseases thrive in an acidic environment and as a result of the mucous build-up in a part of the body and mostly recommended alkaline diet which is usually plant-based. He claims that cells rejuvenation occurs by the elimination of toxic was which happen when the body is being alkalized. He claims that the preference of certain foods and avoidance of some other foods could help to detoxify the body and achieve the state of health necessary to reduce the risk and effects of diseases.

CHAPTER TWO

WHAT IS THE IMMUNE SYSTEM

The immune system is a compound system of cells and proteins that shields the body from all form of infections. The immune system is essential for human survival, as, without it, the body would be an open ground for micro-organism attack without any form of defense. It has a means of identifying any offending germs or microbes it might have previously defended the body against, this helps it to quickly recognize and destroy the microbe if it invades the body again. Humans have three types of immune system; the innate or natural immune system which everybody is born with, the adaptive immune system which is developed over time as man develops and consequently throughout life. The passive immunity is borrowed from another source, and it only lasts for a short time e.g. the immunity of a baby at birth is usually gotten from the mother until the baby immune system is developed enough to fight against invading micro-organism. This is why immunization is very important as it sensitize the baby's immune system to the existence of harmful microorganism and activates it. The main parts of the immune system include: white blood cells also called the leukocytes which include the monocytes, lymphocytes, phagocytes etc., antibodies, the complement system, the lymphatic system, the spleen, the thymus and the bone marrow. All these parts stimulate the body to actively fight against infections. The B- and T-lymphocytes; these are the memory cells of the human immune system. They help to keep records of every microbe the body's immune system has ever destroyed. The white blood cells of the body are the key players in the immune system; they move through the blood and body tissue looking for any invading organism such as bacteria, viruses, parasites, fungi etc. When they find them, they launch an attack against them. The antibodies in the body help to fights against invading microbes in the body and stop the effect of the toxins they produce. The complements cells; as the name implies, is made up of protein that primarily help to balance the effort of the antibodies in the human body. The lymphatic system consists of a network of tubes that are very delicate in the body. They aids to control the fluid levels in the body, reacts violently to bacteria, combat cells products that would otherwise result in initiating diseases in the body and they also absorb some of the body's fats from the intestine. The lymphatic system is made up of the lymphatic nodes, also called lymph glands which re renowned for the ability to rap microorganism, lymph vessels that carry fluid that contains white blood cells.

The spleen, unlike the earlier, mentioned parts of the immune system is a blood-filtering organ that removes microbes from the body and helps to destroy old or damaged red blood cells in the body. The bone marrow is found inside the bone, and it is spongy like in appearance. Its primary purpose is to generate red blood cells that help to circulate oxygen in the body, the white blood cells help the body to fight infections, and the platelet is required by the body for blood clotting in case of an injury. On the other hand, the thymus works like the spleen in filtering and monitoring blood contents, and it produces T-lymphocytes.

CLASSES OF FOOD THAT BOOST THE IMMUNE SYSTEM

There are several classes of food that boost the immune system. But before we get over our selves, I will like to refresh our memories of all the classes of food we have. In basic elementary, it was taught that there are six classes of food which includes; carbohydrates, protein, lipids, vitamins, minerals, and water. Although all these food components contribute their quota to the effectiveness of the body's immune system even if the only minute, there are some of them that work actively to boost the body's immune system. In this group are protein, vitamins are minerals. Other subclasses include; anti-oxidants and anti-inflammatory, flavonoids and carotenoids etc.

WHAT DR. SEBI SAID ABOUT IMMUNITY

Dr Sebi claimed that the immune system is damaged by toxins which in turn increases the susceptibility for infection. He further stressed that acidification from non-natural foods coupled with significant mineral malnutrition could exacerbate issues and significantly affect the body's ability to heal. In addition to this, he said stress and a feeling of fear cause the body to release the hormone that signals immediate danger which in turn causes a reduction in the activity of the body's immune system to preserve energy. This down-regulation has a negative effect on the body as it jeopardizes the defence system against pathogens and microorganism. He then said that if these immune suppressants are eliminated from the body, and the body's nutrition is enhanced, this helps to activate the immune system to keep external threats away from the body. He further describes several Cs that can boost the immune system. They are clean, control, contain, community, calm and care.

Clean: this necessitates the need to wash hands mindfully with soap and water and also wipe surfaces with detergents

Control: this indicates the need to avoid unnecessary gathering and crowds.

Contain: coughs and sneezes should be done in tissues to reduce transmission

Community: this states the need to support the elderly and the children whose immune system are disabled or underdeveloped.

Calm: reduction of stress, need for relaxation, avoiding fear and trusting the body to heal naturally.

Care: this emphasizes the need to adequately look after nutrition and mental wellness and planning how to maintain good health.

He encourages that people should give their immune system the enhancement it needs by detoxifying it through reduction of plastic pesticide, toxin exposure and heavy metals. Purification by staying hydrated with spring water and getting enough iron into the system to maintain the body. He also mentioned restoration and nutrition. Restoration in terms of taking enough rest and getting sufficient sleep for the body. Nutrition by eating alkaline foods and nourishing the body with nature's gift to health.

CHAPTER THREE

ANTI-OXIDANTS AND

ANTI-INFLAMMATORY

The ability of antioxidants to destroy free radicals in the body make them a protector of the structural integrity of cells and tissues in the body. Inflammation though is a natural immune system function, can cause severe damage to the body when it goes out of control. There are some foods that act as anti-inflammatory to prevent this kind of occurrence in the body. Anti-oxidants and anti-inflammatories defend the human cells from the end product of free radicals and reduce the occurrence of the excess of inflammation in the body. Free radicals can cause damage to the DNA, cell membranes and even other parts of the cells. However, these free radicals are void of adequate element electrons, they pinch from other existing molecules and in the process mutilate them. In this effect, anti-oxidants give off their own electrons to the free radicals and prevent them from feeding off the electrons of the body cells thereby preventing damage. Despite the fact that these free radicals are deleterious to health, they are an inescapable part of life. The body tends to generate these free radicals as byproducts of normal cell processes for example when the body's immune system fights an intruder the oxygen it uses in this process produces free radicals that though destroy bacteria and viruses also destroy the body cells. In addition to this, the amount of free radicals increases in response to insults from the environment, such as air pollution, tobacco smoke, ultraviolet rays. This is why anti-oxidants are very important in the body. The free radicals are so pervasive that an adequate supply of anti-oxidants is needed to disarm them. Though the body cells produce some level of anti-oxidants, the anti-oxidants gotten from food are of great importance.

BENEFITS

- They help the body to fight against free radicals.-

- It reduces the risk for diseases or infection

- It scavenges free radicals from the body cells

- It protects the body against cell damage

- It minimizes reactions that cause excessive inflammation in the body.

MEAL TIPS

Some of these anti-oxidants include

Hesperetin which is found in oranges and other citrus fruits. They help to restore vitamin C to its active anti-oxidant form after it has given its electron to a free radical. Others include; Anthocyanins, lycopene, flavanols, catechins, kaempferol, isothiocyanates, polyphenols, quercetin, lignin, indoles, lutein etc. are examples of anti-oxidants.

Some natural foods that contain these anti-oxidants are beets, blueberries, broccoli, onion, garlic, turmeric, dark chocolate, pumpkin, kiwi fruits, grapes, mangoes, spinach, sesame seeds, peas, nuts, milk, cabbage, soybeans, bran, thyme, oregano, tomatoes, watermelon etc.

OMEGA -3 FATTY ACIDS, FLAVONOIDS, AND MINERALS

Omega 3-fatty acids are essential fatty acids that are renowned for their role in helping to maintain the cell membrane of the body. Aside from this, they play a very crucial role in regulating the gene expression of white blood cells which in turn regulates proper immune function in the body. The body's cell membrane is a wall between the internal cell content and the environments. The cell membrane helps the cell to hold water as well as other nutrients that are needed for cell survival. Research has shown that cell membranes are composed of fatty acids which can be derived from diets rich in omega 3-fatty acids. Omega 3-fatty acids reduce the production of anti-inflammatory compounds that causes damages to the immune system. It also plays an important role in helping to improve the communication between the immune system, thereby enhancing their activity and leading to an improved immune system. Omega 3s has been known to have a profound effect on the body prostaglandin and as such helps them to properly mediate physiological processes in the body and makes them abundantly useful in virtually every state of diseases. Many kinds of research have also shown that omega 3- fats stimulate the proliferation of T-cells. The adequate functionality of T cells is vital to our immune system as we have earlier ascertained that T cells form a significant part of the body's immune system.

BENEFITS

- Omega-3 fights long term inflammation by reducing and substances associated with inflammation such as cytokines and eicosanoids

- It helps to fight autoimmune diseases which happen when the body mistakes normal healthy cells for f5oreign cells and work to attack them.

- It helps in adequate maintenance of body cells.

MEAL TIP

Example of food rich in omega-3 fatty acids are

Omega -3: flax seed, seaweed, salmon fish, tuna, lake trout, blue fish, halibut, striped bass, eggs, soy beans, spinach, cod liver oil, caviar, mackerel, anchovies, chia seeds, peanut butter, almonds, pumpkin seeds, Hemp seeds, walnuts, mung beans, cabbage.

FLAVONOIDS

Flavonoids are considered as plants secondary metabolites, and they have numerous effects on the immune system. They belong to the group of naturally occurring phenylchromones in plants. They function as anti-oxidants, anti-mutagenic, antibacterial, anti-allergy, enzyme modulation, and anticancer. Fruits, vegetables, grains, barks, roots, stems, flowers, and tea are good sources of flavonoids. Flavonoids alongside carotenoids are responsible for the vivid colours in fruits. Flavonoids have 6,000 variants which make it the largest group of phytonutrients. The several significant groups of flavonoids include; flavanols, flavones, flavonols, flavonones and isoflavone. Each of these originating groups carries their own set of actions as they contain different phytochemicals.

BENEFITS

- They help to destroy free radicals that can damage the body cells

- They act as anti-histamine which allows to control the release of histamine in the body thereby reducing the abundance of inflammations and other symptoms

- It has anti-microbial property which makes it effective in helping the body o fight against invading bacteria in the body.

- It helps to modulate lipid peroxidation, thereby reducing low-density lipoproteins in the body.

MEAL TIP

Example of foods found in this group are celery, parsley, hot peppers, grapes, pomegranate, soy beans, legumes, Brussels sprout, kale, berries, apples, green tea, chamomile tea, nuts oranges, lemon, cherry etc.

SELENIUM

Selenium is one of the minerals that the body seems to benefit gravely from. It has both structural and enzymatic roles which makes it more effective in helping to boost the immune system and slow down the body's overactive responses. It also helps to lower the body's oxidative stress and is a crucial nutrient in counteracting the development of virulence. It is found in Brazil nuts, barley, tuna, sea foods, egg, brown rice, bananas, lentils, cashews etc.

ZINC

Zinc is very crucial in the development and proper functioning of cells that mediate innate immunity and neutrophils. Studies have shown that insufficient zinc in the body has an adverse effect of the macrophages, which forms part of the body's defense system. The rate at which phagocytosis occurs, the growth and function of T and B cells and the rate of cytokine production are known to be affected by zinc deficiency. They also have an anti-oxidant property which gives them the ability to counteract the body's free radicals. Examples of foods that are rich in zinc are meat, shellfish, legumes, dairy products, eggs, dark chocolate etc.

Phosphorus is another mineral that contributes to immune system health as it plays important role in bone formation, energy metabolism, cellular signaling and stabilization of cell membranes. Other minerals that help to boost the immune system include magnesium, sulphur (allicin compounds) etc.

VITAMINS A, C, B-6, D, E

VITAMIN A

This is a class of micronutrient that plays an impressive role in boosting the human immune system. Vitamin A contains caretenoids which have an antioxidant effect and plays an important role in strengthening the immune system to fight against infectious diseases. Over time, vitamin A has proven itself to be essential for the development of tissues that protect human against pathogens and harmful microorganism. It provides humans with a highly functional immune system which is the essence of good health. It also provides the energy that is needed for the body's homeostasis most especially the homeostasis of the bone marrow by normal apostosis processes of bone marrow cells. It plays an important role in helping human growth and development and it has anti-inflammatory ability there preventing overabundance of inflammation that can damage the body cells. Study has shown that crucial organs of the immune system need enough dose of vitamin A to proliferate, differentiate, mature, aggregate and respond as expected. It helps to maintain the functional and structural membranes of the mucosal lining of the body and is responsible for the generation of antibody that responds to specific antigens in the body.

BENEFITS

- They maintain the normal defences in the body.

- They help to protect the mucous membrane in the eyes, lungs and genitals which serves as a barrier that helps the body to trap invading microorganism.

- It is involved in the production and efficient functioning of the body's white blood cells.

- It plays an active role in cell differentiation and maintenance of epithelial surfaces.

MEAL TIPS

Examples of food in which vitamin A can be found are liver, carrot, cod-liver oil, butter, eggs, spinach, vegetables, sweet potatoes, cantaloupe, squash, broccoli, grape etc.

VITAMIN C

Vitamin C is an essential micronutrient that has lots of advantage in the immune system. It is well known for its ability to donate electrons to antioxidants after they donate theirs to free radical in the bodies. This helps the antioxidants to return to its original state in preparation to make another donate when a new free radical appears. Aside from this, vitamin C has been known to acts as an antioxidant itself, and they contribute immensely to biosynthesis and gene regulation. It supports the cellular functions of both innate and adaptive immune system, which is one of its significant contribution to the immune defense. Studies have shown that vitamin C supports the epithelial tissues lining the barriers of the body which make them function optimally against pathogens and microorganisms and also protects the body again environmental oxidative stress by promoting the oxidant scavenging activity of the skin. It enhances chemotaxis, phagocytosis, species of reactive oxygen generation and microbial killing. Over time, vitamin C has been used medically for the treatment of respiratory and systemic infections. Prophylactically, it produces adequate, if not saturating plasma levels which gives the body the needed boost against infections. Vitamin C, also known as ascorbic acid, is not produced by the body but is gotten from food and fruits, which is the more reason it must be included in food regimen.

BENEFITS

- It is a powerful antioxidant that strengthens the body's immune system and the body's natural defence's.

- It enhances the production of white blood cells and phagocytes which are needed to fight against invading microorganisms

- It is responsible for the growth and repair of damaged tissue by shortening the time needed for wound healing and contributing actively to the wound healing process.

- It supports the production of interferons which are produced in the detection of pathogens and turn facilitate the cell involved to initiate protective cellular defence's

- It enhances cytokine production of the white blood cells and inhibits the apoptosis of T-lymphocytes.

- It plays an active role in the inhibition of neuraminidase, an enzyme that keeps viruses and

bacterial l trapped in the mucosa
lining in the body.

- It inhibits histamine and supports the
production of prostaglandin and
antibodies in the body.

- It enhances the mucolytic effect by
turning fatty acids into fluids, thereby
increasing the access of the body's
immune system to invading pathogens
and makes the bacterial membrane
more permeable to antibiotics, thus
decreasing their viability.

MEAL TIPS

Given the fact that vitamin C is not
made by the body and has to vet
gotten from good external products, it

is good news that sources of vitamin C are abundant. Some of which includes: oranges, grapefruit, brussels sprouts, broccoli, green and red bell pepper, tomatoes, strawberries, kiwi fruit, cauliflower, spinach, cabbage, turnip greens, sweet potatoes, pawpaw, kale, cantaloupe and many more.

VITAMIN B-6

It has been earlier established that B and T lymphocytes contribute greatly to the activities of the immune system by helping to keep a record of all the disease the system has attacked which makes the immune system better ready to fight such disease when they come invading again. Vitamin B6 known less commonly as pyridoxine contributes greatly to the production of these white blood cells and helps to regulate their functions, making them respond as appropriate when needed. This vitamin is also a major contributor to the production of a protein called interleukin-2 which helps to direct the actions of white blood cells in this body-enhancing their ability to fight disease. Vitamin B6 contributes greatly in helping to produce antibodies that fight against infections and also helps the body to make enough haemoglobin needed for carrying oxygen to the required organs in the body. Studies have shown that the deficiency of vitamin B6 on the body affects both the homoral and the cell-mediated responses of the immune system. Vitamin B6 helps in the differentiation and maturation of the body lymphocytes, enhances the body's responses to a hypersensitivity reaction and increases the production of antibodies to combat infections.

BENEFITS

- It helps the body to process homocysteine which is a byproduct of protein metabolism and the high availability of it in the body can lead to several diseases.

- It supports biochemical reactions that occur in the immune system and as a result, promotes its ability to protect the body against invading pathogens and microorganisms.

- It actively contributes to the removal of unwanted chemicals that are deleterious to the body system.

- It contributes greatly to the body's coenzymatic activity and improves metabolism, all of which are needed for the adequate function of the immune system.

- It refurbishes the body's immune system to its required functional state which helps it to withstand numerous kinds of infections.

- It increases the level of prostaglandin in the body, thereby reducing susceptibility to diseases and infections.

MEAL TIP

Examples of food rich in vitamin B6 are; lentils, banana, Brussel sprouts, avocado, prunes, spinach, soya beans, liver, beef, pork, tuna, milk, salmon, eggs, fish, sunflower seeds, nuts, vegetables, bran among many others.

VITAMIN D

The deficiency of vitamin D is very common nowadays as the major source of vitamin D is sunlight and people keep reducing their exposure to this sunlight on a daily basis. The very few who do wears toxic sunscreen which prevents the skin from getting the necessary sun rays needed to synthesize vitamin D. More so; technology has made it so people who aren't working from home can stay in the coolness of their car or service with minimal exposure to sunlight. In addition to this, not many foods are naturally rich in vitamin D which makes its unavailability by shying away from the sun very difficult to make up for. This has made the deficiency of vitamin D to be on the increase. It works tirelessly to help activate processes that the body need to maintain health. It reduces the risk of infection by strengthening the innate immune system of the body. Vitamin D has been known to use peptides to trigger antimicrobial responses in the body, thereby inhibiting the effect of bacteria and prevent a full-blown infection.

BENEFITS

- It helps to prevent autoimmune disease by regulating the T cells and teaching the body to identify its own cell thereby preventing an attack against them.

- It helps to destroy chemicals that kills the body's native tissue.

- It acts as an anti-inflammatory and helps to reduce inflammation to prevent its overabundance.

- It helps to maintain healthy bone and teeth since it regulates the absorption of calcium needed for the growth of bone and teeth in the body.

- Vitamin D works actively in the mission of the body to fight against diseases.

MEAL TIP

As earlier mentioned, vitamin D is not very much available naturally in foods and fruits because just like vitamin K, it is one of the very few vitamins the body synthesizes on its own. Even though in low quantity, it can still be found in food products like fish, especially fatty fish such as tuna, salmon, mackerel etc., Liver, cheese, egg yolks, mushrooms, almond, cereals, tofu, cheese, oatmeal etc.

VITAMIN E

Vitamin E also called Tocopherol, is a micronutrient that acts as an antioxidant that protects the body against free radicals. It helps to modulate immune functions in such a way that the defense system is active enough to diseases and infections. It is usually found in higher concentration in the immune system than other parts of the body. It has a direct impact on the T cells of the immune system, signal transduction, membrane integrity and cell division which are processes that helps to maintain the body's homeostasis. It also has an indirect impact on inflammatory mediators. Previously conducted studies have shown that vitamin E contributes immensely to the production of interferons and interleukins that strengthens the immune system, in turn, strengthening its ability to fight against infection. Vitamin E presents free radicals the electrons they need, which in turn prevent the radicals from feeding off of the electrons of the body cells.

BENEFITS

- It enhances T cells activation and functionality.

- It aids to generate prostaglandin.

- It protects body cells from damage.

- It shields the body from oxidative damage.

- It gives extra protection to the body cells, especially this did the immune system.

- It helps in the structural and functional maintenance of skeletal cardiac and smooth muscles.

- it helps in healing and prevents excessive scar formation.

- It contributes enormously to cardiovascular health by keeping the arteries healthy and working as a blood thinner which prevents the formation of clots by blood platelets in the blood vessels. These clots can easily cause TIA or stroke.

MEAL TIPS

Vitamin E is available in many forms of food and fruits some of which includes; hazelnuts, peanuts, almond, spinach, broccoli, mango, kiwi fruit, tomatoes, avocado, kale, sunflower seeds, parsley, turnip greens, Swiss chards, mustard, papaya, green olive, bell pepper, dry apricots, chilli

powder, cereals, seafood among many
others.

CONCLUSION

Having read through the book, I hope you have been able to learn about the classes of food that contributes towards the health of the immune system. The role they play and how each of them can singly or collaboratively perform its function in boosting the body's immune system. The fact is we are what we eat as this reflects directly on our health, emotions and even daily activities. I very much wish you will put the knowledge you have gained into action and start feeding your body food that will aid the activities of its immune system, and he'll you to stay healthy. Best of luck!

www.ingramcontent.com/pod-product-compliance
Lightning Source LLC
Chambersburg PA
CBHW051233250726
48655CB00006B/2746